Mint, the Miraculous Herb

And more than 30 ways to use it

More books by Evelyn Key:

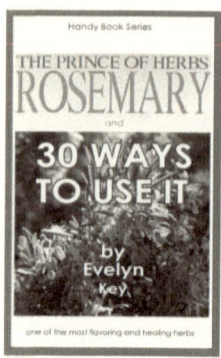
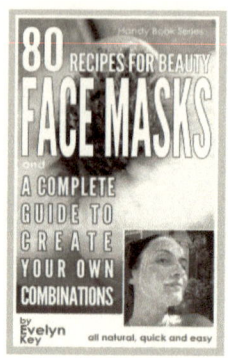

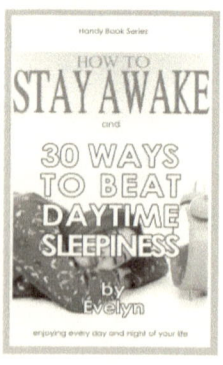
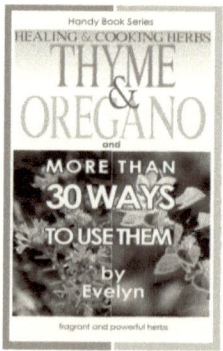

Mint, the Miraculous Herb
And more than 30 ways to use it

Evelyn Key

Handy Book Series
2014

Mint, the Miraculous Herb

First Printing: 2014

ISBN 978-1-312-62229-6

Evaggelia Karageorge
P.O. 1866, Agios Spyridon, Porto Rafti
Markopoulo, Attica, Greece, 19003

Handy Book Series
evelinbooks.wordpress.com
evelynbooks@gmail.com

Dedication

To all the optimist, happy and devoted people of this planet!

You create your life, you create the world!

Contents

Introduction ………………………………………….... 7

Cautions ………………………………………… 10

The Basics ……………………………………… 11

Mint Properties and Benefits ………………………… 14

When it bites or burns …………………………… 15

It's all in my head… ...……………………………… 17

Belly Talks… …………………………………… 19

She's fresh… exciting! ………………………… 21

The Beauty and the… Mint! ……………………….. 25

You take my pain away… …………………………... 29

A "minty" touch in my kitchen… …………………… 31

Mint Varieties ………………………………….. 35

Just a few mint quotes before you go… ……………… 37

References and Notes ………………………….. 38

Disclaimer ……………………………………… 40

Reviews ………………………………………… 42

Introduction

"Mint the miraculous herb, and more than 30 Ways to use it," presents the wondrous world of mint, probably the most famous herb around the world and through history! Actually, certain references in Linear B scripts (1), about mint storage methods and perfume manufacturing, indicate its presence, at least, since the Minoan Age.

Over the centuries, mint has often been called as the "oldest medicine in the world" or "the miraculous herb," while, nowadays, continues to hold the place of the most popular herb.

There are at least 30 kinds of mint, and they all belong to the "Labiatae"(2) family of aromatic herbs. However, two specific varieties stand out among the others because these are the most used worldwide. They have similar properties and people often confuse the one with the other:

I'm referring to **Spearmint** (Mentha Spicata syn. Mentha Viridis) and **Peppermint** (Mentha Piperita.) Peppermint is a hybrid, derived from the crossing between Mentha Aquatica and Mentha Spicata. This book is dedicated to these two species of mint and their uses.

In Greece, spearmint is the most common kind of mint. The Greek name of spearmint is *"Diosmos"* and it means "**Sweet Scent.**"

THE MYTH OF MINT comes from the ancient Greek Mythology, and the name Mint is derived from"**Minthe.**"

Minthe was one of the Naiads, the nymphs who lived in the county of Elis in Greece. She was the daughter of Kokytos (3), and her beauty was so marvellous that **Pluto**, the God of the underworld, fell in love with her. He first saw her wandering in the woods of the highest mountain in the province of Olympia, in Greece; later, this mountain was named after her. Pluto, dazzled by her beauty, decided that he had to make her his mistress.

According to one version of the myth, Persephone, Pluto's wife, saw him kissing Minthe, and she told her mother, the goddess Demeter. The Goddess punished Minthe by transforming her into a plant, so small and subtle that could be easily stepped on. Pluto, grieving for Minthe, endowed the plant with an exceptional scent.

Another variant of the myth, says that Demeter herself trampled on Minthi, and Pluto didn't defend her. He just transformed her into a fragrant plant, which began to grow on the slopes of the mountain Minthi.

There are also other versions, saying that Persephone was the one who trampled on the poor Minthe.

Strabo, a traveller of 175 AD, writes: "*East of Pylos there is a mountain named Minthe, that the legend says she was a mistress of Hades (Pluto) and she was trampled by the young lady, so the Minthe turned into the garden Minthe, that some call mint.*"

This myth explains why mint and its wonderful aroma, was dedicated to the god Pluto (Hades).

AROUND THE WORLD AND THROUGH HISTORY

The ancient Greeks believed that mint refreshes the mind, cures headaches and cools the blood. It is said that they were wearing wreaths of mint on their heads after wine drinking, to avoid headache symptoms. They were also used it for body rejuvenation and hiccups soothing.

The admiration of mint was quite common in ancient Rome as well. The Romans flavoured their food with mint leaves, and washed their bodies with mint scented water.

In the Middle Ages, monks use it both in cooking and healing remedies.

Furthermore, mint is vastly beloved and praised in the Arab world, that people use to swear in the name of it. Its Arabic name means "gift of Allah" (naana).

The Chinese used the wild mint of fields since the ancient times (Mentha Arvensis, Bo-He)

In Europe, the cultivation of mint was developed after the 18th century, when the English began to grow it in the outskirts of London.

FEATURES AND CULTIVATION

Mint can withstand high temperatures as long as it is watered quite often, about 3-4 times a week. It needs moisture. The optimum growth temperature for the mint is at 17oC.

Nevertheless, it thrives in hot and dry climates as well as in lowland areas and fertile grounds.

It is propagated by cuttings, planted during the autumn months. Roots, on the other hand, are best to be planted in the spring.

Mint blooms in early July and its flowers have white or violet colour.

Some basic differences between spearmint and peppermint, are the following:

-The stem of spearmint is green while the peppermint's reddish.

-The leaves of spearmint have more intense nerves than peppermint's.

-The peppermint leaves colour is slightly darker and greener than spearmint.

The ingredients, and their levels, vary among the different varieties of mint.

It contains: Menthol (alcohol), menthone (ketone), tannins. The leaves of peppermint contain vitamins A, C and niacin.

COLLECT AND USE

The useful parts of the plant are the leaves and the flowering tops. There are two periods for collecting: first in July, at the beginning of the flowering, and secondly, in the early autumn. Always make sure that you do not to collect excessive amounts; store only as much as you need until the next season.

The dry mint loses almost the 70% of its aroma.

Six hundred pounds of mint leaves are needed, to extract two litres of essential oil.

Mint is widely used in cooking, wine and pharmaceutical products. Yet, nowadays, the massive production of the industrial products, often uses synthetic fragrance instead of the original mint essential oil.

Cautions

- Avoid mint during breastfeeding.
- Children should not take it for longer than a week.
- Do not give mint, in any form, to infants.
- The **essential oil** of mint should not be used by epileptics, pregnant women, nursing and young children.
- In any case of special medical conditions, always consult your doctor first.

The Basics

In this chapter is an introduction to the basic formulations that can be prepared at home, and used in various purposes.

Tincture

Tincture is the alcoholic extract of an herb. (Alcohol 35-90% by volume). Several alcoholic ethanol solutions can be used as well, such as vodka, white rum (alcohol 40-50%) or even strong apple cider vinegar.

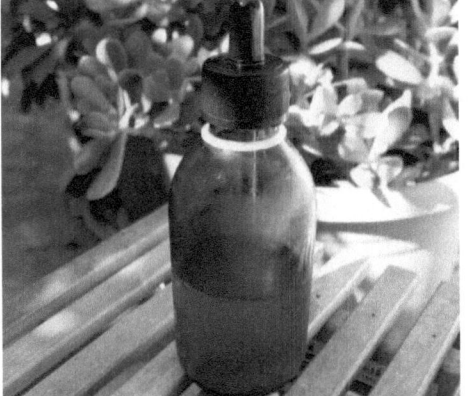

DOSAGE:
A handful of mint
1 cup of alcohol
PREPARATION: Cut the leaves of mint; use your hands rather than metal objects such as knives. Put the leaves in a glass or ceramic jar with a lid; no metal parts. Mash the leaves a bit with a ceramic pestle. Pour the alcohol, close the jar and shake slightly.

Keep it in a shady place for almost one month, shaking once a day or every other day. Thereafter, strain and store in a dark glass bottle, with a dropper on the cap if possible.

The dropper is very handy, since you will be using only a few drops of this formulation.

Mint oil

Mint oil is the mint infusion in a plant oil such as almond, Jojoba, sesame or even olive oil. However, in cases of external use, lighter and odourless oils are the best choice.
DOSAGE:
4 Oz almond oil
1 cup fresh mint leaves

PREPARATION: Place the mint leaves in a glass jar with a lid. Pour in the oil and close well. Shake and let it in a sunny place for almost twenty days. Shake the jar once a day and check for signs of moisture and mould inside the lid. After twenty days, remove the mint leaves and store it in a dark glass bottle.

A cup of mint

DECOTION: you may use the fresh flowering tops and the leaves of the plant.Mint stimulates the blood circulation and increases the body's temperature.

Prepare a mint decoction by boiling 3 teaspoons of mint leaves/flowers in 2 cups of water, for 3-5 minutes. Remove from heat and strain into a cup.

INFUSION: Heat the water and remove from fire just before it comes to a boil. In a teapot or a cup, put the mint leaves and pour the hot water (1 teaspoon of dry leaves for each cup of water). Cover and let it stand for half an hour. Strain.

Do not exceed 1-2 cups a day, for a period up to 2 months; avoid mint if you are on homeopathic therapy.

Poultice (Cataplasm)

Following the same procedure, you can prepare a poultice of any other herb.

DRIED MINT: Crush the dried mint leaves with a pestle or rub it with your finger. Add a few drops of warm water, enough to make a paste.

Notes: Warm apple vinegar is also proper to use.

Apply this paste directly to the hurting body part. As the poultice dries, the skin absorbs the therapeutic substances of the mint.

Another way to apply the poultice, is this: on a gauze pad, spread a layer of the mint paste, put one more gauze above it, and place it on the traumatized spot.

FRESH MINT: In a pot, add ½ cup of water and ½ cup mint leaves and let it simmer, until a thick mass is left. Apply as above.

Important: Keep the poultices warm. When you feel the pain subside, then the poultice has done its job!

Water for bathing

Boil 2 litres of water (about 8 ½ cups.) Remove from the fire and allow to cool just for a while; 3-4 minutes, depending on environmental temperature.

Add about 6 tablespoons of dried mint and let it stand for 1 hour. Strain.

You can add this infusion to your bath water, or make a foot bath, soak your hands or even rinse your hair after shampooing.

Store in the refrigerator for one week maximum. Warm it before use, but beware not to boil.

Mint Properties and Benefits

"For someone to name all the properties of mint, must know how many fish swim in the Indian Ocean" Naturalist of the 12th century

- Accelerates the heart rate
- Aphrodisiac
- Analgesic
- Antibacterial
- Antiemetic (Stops vomiting)
- Antipyretic
- Antiseptic
- Antispasmodic
- Anxiety
- Asthma
- Bronchitis
- Burns
- Calming
- Cough and sore throat
- Disinfectant
- Diuretic
- Dizziness
- Expectorant
- Headaches
- Heart diseases
- Increases body temperature
- Indigestion
- Insomnia
- Liver function
- Memory
- Mood elevator
- Muscle contractions
- Nervous disorders
- Oral and throat infections
- Rheumatism
- Stimulates the production of bile
- Stomach and digestive system (stomach cramps, aerophagy, bloating, nausea)
- Tremors

When it bites or burns

Mint is a proper remedy for insect or reptile bites, as well as for other skin irritations such as burns.

Apart from its healing properties, mint scent is repulsive for some animals, like mice that can't withstand it.

Bites from insects and reptiles

Mint remedies can relieve the pain from stings and bites. However, in cases of poisonous stings and bites or if you have any allergies, medical care is mandatory.

SOOTHING OIL: Blend 2 drops of mint essential oil with 1 tbsp olive oil. Apply the mixture on the bite; it will soothe the pain and the irritation.

Alternatively, you can use some homemade mint oil extract (page 11).

MINT TINCTURE: Apply with a cotton pad on the hurting spot and keep it there for a few minutes.

CATAPLASM: Use a pestle to crush the mint leaves with 1 tbsp salt. Add a few drops of distilled water and make a paste. Apply it as a poultice on the bite.

REPELLENT: To repel mosquitoes, rub some mint leaves on your skin.

Burns

For mild minor burns and pain relief, prepare:
- A mint poultice, to relieve the pain of burns (page 12)
- Apply a layer of homemade mint oil extract (page 11)
- Prepare a mint infusion, add 2 drops of mint essential oil (optional) and shake. Put it in a spray bottle and refresh your body after sunbathing.

Mint, the Miraculous Herb

It's all in my head...

Dizziness, headaches, migraines

Hippocrates and Galinos used mint against vertigo and headaches (4,5). It was considered as one of the most ideal remedies for the pains of the head.

POULTICE: American Indians, and other ancient or primitive cultures around the world, used to chew herbs to make a liquid pulp. Then, they applied this pulp as a poultice on the hurting body parts.

- Prepare a poultice (pag.12) with mint leaves and place it on the forehead. When the herb comes in contact with the skin, the body absorbs its healing properties. You can use fresh or dried mint.
- Crush 10 fresh mint leaves along with a slice of lemon and use this mixture as a poultice.
- Relax with a mint poultice on your forehead, while you drink a mint tea with lemon!
- A simpler, alternative, way is to rub peppermint leaves on the forehead.

MINT OIL: Massage your forehead, temples and back of your neck with mint oil extract.

RELAXING BEVERAGE: Drink a relaxing chamomile infusion mixed with 10 drops of mint tincture.

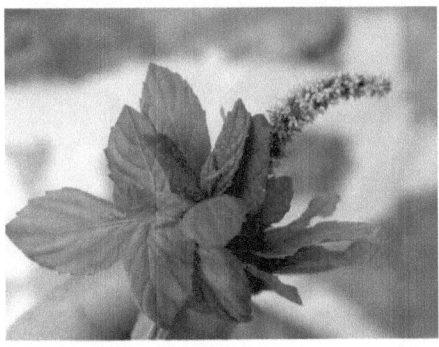

Nervous and mental disorders

Menthol's muscle relaxant properties may be particularly helpful in cases of anxiety [6].

Mint scent has the ability to repel negative thoughts.

In aromatherapy, peppermint essential oil is used in cases of mental fatigue and depression. It is very beneficial since it elevates the mood and banishes fears.

- **A mint tea** (decoction or infusion) could be very calming for nervous disorders, which are manifested by dry cough, trouble sleeping, etc.
- Say yes to a nice **massage with peppermint oil!** You can use the homemade oil extract (pag.11) or a mixture of almond oil with peppermint essential oil: 2 drops essential oil/1 tablespoon of almond oil.
- Have a cloth **handkerchief, scented with mint** essential oil, always in your pocket, and smell it whenever your mood needs an uplift.

Belly Talks...

Sexual impotence

The aphrodisiac properties of this herb, have been highly praised since the ancient era.

In the Arab world, mint, and specifically peppermint tea, have been used to enhance the sexual arousal; a tradition derived from antiquity.

Even Shakespeare mentions mint as a stimulant for men of any age, in combination with lavender and rosemary. (The Winter's Tale)

It is said that Aristotle advised Alexander the Great to prohibit his soldiers from drinking mint tea before the battle, in order to avoid sexual arousal and the subsequent loss of their force.

- Use an essential oil diffuser to fragrance your space with mint scent.
- Serve a cup of strong mint tea or a portion of mint liqueur.

Caution: Large quantities of mint tea may cause the opposite results.

Indigestion (7)

Ingredients:
1 tbsp fresh ginger
1 handful fresh spearmint
1 kiwi
1 cup pineapple
Put the above ingredients in a juice extractor and drink their valuable juice.

Stomach tonic

Mint has been used for indigestion issues since the era of Hippocrates and Galinos. Dioscorides have said that mint is friendly to the stomach, while Plinios writes: *".. It calms the stomach pain and removes intestinal parasites"*

The antispasmodic properties of menthol, relieve the stomach disorders. The clinical administration of peppermint oil has been shown to help people who suffer from Irritable Bowel Syndrome (IBS) (8).

- **A decoction or infusion** of mint can help: Indigestion, Diarrhoea, Intestinal inflammations, After vomiting (pennyroyal.)
- **Three drops of mint** essential oil in a glass of water after meals relieves indigestion, colic and facilitates expulsion of stomach gas.
- **It is said that the combination** of mint with cumin essential oil also relieves acid indigestion; 2 drops of each in a glass of water.

She's fresh... exciting!

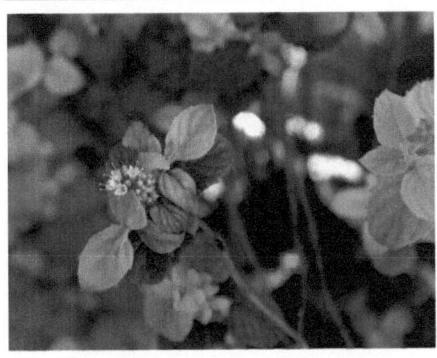

The first references about teeth cleaning creams, with mint ingredient, have been found in scripts of the 6th century AC.

Cut and chew some mint leaves and feel the sense of pure freshness in your mouth!

Mouth and throat diseases

Mint is ideal for bad breath, since it fights germs of teeth and gums. Not only freshens the breath, but gargling with essential oil and water helps also in cases of tonsillitis, oral cavity or throat inflammation, and gum disease.

Liquid mixtures for Gargling:
- Add 8 drops of peppermint essential oil in a glass of distilled water.
- Add a few drops of mint tincture (pag.11) in a cup of mint infusion.

Mouthwash recipes

If you like the idea of a homemade mouthwash, here are a few recipes to try:

Recipe-A:
- 2 cups of rose water or green tea
- 10 drops of peppermint essential oil
- 5 drops of lemon essential oil

In a sterilized bottle, add the flower water or green tea and the essential oils. Shake well and use as a mouthwash.

You can store it in the fridge. Do not buy green tea in ready to drink packs, because they contain chemical additives; always prepare it yourself.

Recipe B:
2 cups distilled water
1 teaspoon mint
1 teaspoon rosemary
Mint tincture

Prepare the infusion and let it chill. Then, add 10 drops of mint tincture. Shake and rinse your mouth. Store in the refrigerator. Both rosemary and mint, have antiseptic properties.

Recipe C:
1 cup distilled water
7 drops of peppermint essential oil
1 teaspoon baking soda

In a sterilized bottle, with a large nozzle and a cap, add 1 cup of water and the essential oil. Shake well. Add the baking soda, close the cap and shake again. Rinse your mouth and keep the rest in the refrigerator for later use. Always shake before use.

Toothpaste

"One drachma of rock salt, two drachmas of mint, one drachma of dried iris flower and 20 grains of pepper, all of them crushed and mixed together." (11)

Ingredients
3 tsp of baking soda (organic)
1 tsp ground sea salt
1 tsp stevia sweetener
1 tbsp ground dried mint
10 drops of mint essential oil
3 tsp plant glycerine or 2-3 tbsp coconut oil

Preparation: Use a coffee grinder to grind the sea salt and the dried mint. Put the powder mixture in a small bowl, add the stevia and the baking soda, and mix well.

Then add the glycerine or the coconut oil* and the mint essential oil. Mix very well the ingredients to unify, and the homemade toothpaste, is ready for use.

*melt it with the bain marrie method (double boiler.)

Armpits deodorant

The deodorizing properties of mint were recognized since the ancient years.

What could be better than a natural body deodorant, free of chemicals and toxic elements?

Ingredients
1 lemon
5 tbsp mint infusion
2 drops mint essential oil
2 tsp rubbing alcohol
How to: Put the lemon juice and the rest of the ingredients in a small bottle and shake. Let it stand for 2 days before use.

Keep it in a spray or roll on bottle. If you have such bottles from old deodorants, clean them well and sterilize.

Mint, the Miraculous Herb

The Beauty and the... Mint!

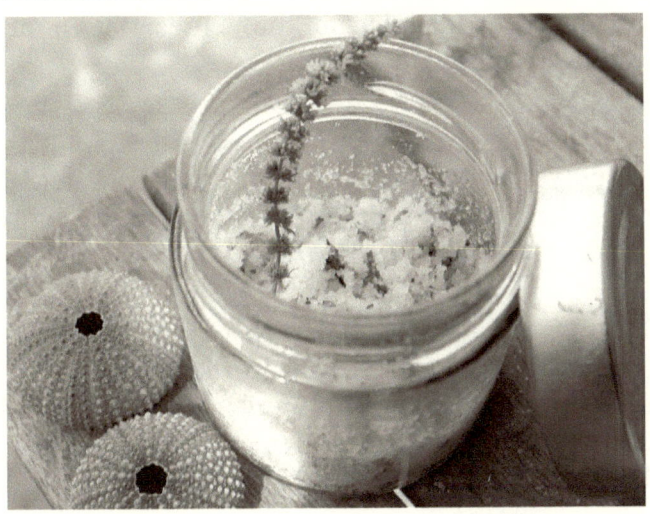

Bathing

The Ancient Greeks, and later the Romans, used to fragrance their bathing water with mint.

If you like to try it, prepare mint bathing water as described on page , and if you want to enhance its power, add:

- 15 drops of mint essential oil, **or**
- Bath salts mixed with mint essential oil.

Face mask

The antibacterial and refreshing properties of mint, compose an effective body cleansing that soothes and revitalizes the skin.

The following mask recipe nourishes the dull skin and improves oiliness.

Ingredients

A handful of fresh mint leaves

1 egg yolk

½ cucumber

1 tsp of lemon juice.

How to: In a blender, add the mint leaves, the egg yolk and the cucumber, and blend. Pour the mixture in a bowl, add the lemon juice and stir to unify. Apply on clean and warm skin. Rinse and re-move after 10-15 minutes, with lukewarm water at first and then cold.

Apart from its disinfectant properties, the mint refreshes, stimulates and cleans the skin deeply.

Skin lotion

In a sprayer bottle, put 2 cups of distilled water, 10 drops of mint oil and 10 drops of mint tincture. Shake well and spray your skin whenever it needs a touch of freshness and rejuvenation.

Dandruff and lice

It is said that mint removes dandruff and lice.

Boil a mixture of 1 cup of water, 1 cup of apple cider vinegar and a handful of fresh mint leaves. Remove the leaves and let it chill. Massage the scalp and do not rinse.

Lotion for oily hair

This lotion balances the scalp oiliness.

Ingredients:

2 tbsp fresh mint leaves

2 tbsp rosemary

1 cup of boiled water

How to: Boil the water and remove from fire. Pour the hot water over the herbs, and let it stand for 20 minutes. Strain.

Add 2 tbsp of the lotion in ¼ cup of shampoo. Mix very well to unify completely. Massage your scalp while washing your hair and let it act for a few minutes before rinsing. For best results, use a mild, gentle and organic shampoo.

Another option is to massage your scalp with a small portion of the lotion, after shampooing and rinsing.

Hair mask

Ingredients:

1 ripe banana

10 drops of peppermint essential oil

1 tbsp coconut milk

½ tsp sweet almond oil

Preparation:

In a blender or in a bowl: mash the banana, add the oils and the coconut milk and unify until it gets a creamy texture. Before shampooing, apply the mask on your hair and massage gently. Let it stay for about 20 minutes. Shampoo and rinse well.

Lip balm

How about a homemade lip balm? The peppermint essential oil improves blood circulation and therefore is a fine ingredient for a stimulating lip balm.

Ingredients:

1-2 tbsp coconut oil or cocoa butter

1 tsp honey

5 drops of mint essential oil

Preparation:

Put the coconut oil or the cocoa butter in a tiny glass vase; you could use one of an old lip balm. Warm it with the Bain Marie method, until the coconut oil or the cocoa butter melts. Remove from fire, add the mint essential oil and the honey and mix to unify. Let it cool down. Your homemade lip balm is ready!

Eye compresses-mask

A refreshing, quick and easy mask for your eyes only!

Ingredients:

1 green tea bag

1 cup of water

10 leaves of fresh mint

2 cotton pads

Preparation:

Prepare a cup of green tea. You can drink most of it because you need only a small portion.

Chop the mint leaves.

Dip the cotton pads in the tea, and press them with your fingers to remove most liquids. Lay back and spread the chopped mint leaves around your eyes and put the cotton tabs on top. Stay there for about 15 minutes.

Body scrub

A cool and refreshing, but most of all, natural body scrub!

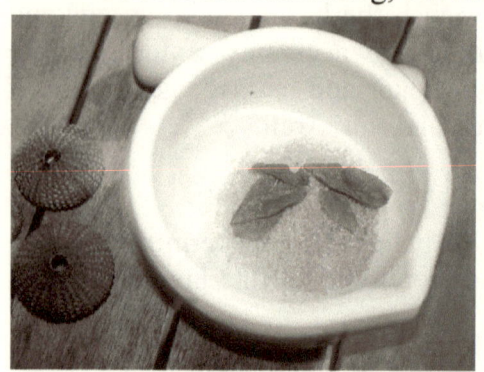

Ingredients:
4 tbsp raw cane sugar
3 tbsp olive, almond or sesame oil
5 drops of mint essential oil or 10 fresh mint leaves

How to:
Put the sugar in a bowl or in a glass jar and crush it a little with a pestle. Add the oils and mix very well. Apply the scrub on clean skin and rinse. Keep the rest in the fridge.

If you use fresh leaves, put them in the bowl with the sugar and crush them together. Then, add the oil and mix.

After a nice bath, while your skin is still fresh, take small portions of the mixture and scrub gently; especially the parts that need it the most, like elbows, knees and heels. Rinse well and wipe gently with a soft towel. Apply a moisturizing body cream, or better yet, a natural oil.

You take my pain away...

All the scientific writings of pharmacology, until the 2nd World War, were almost exclusively filled with herbal remedies. Even if herbs were referred by their scientific names, herbal medications remained the same through the centuries up to modern times.

The demand for drugs was increased dramatically during the war period, and afterwards, the pharmaceutical industry followed the path of chemistry. These changes were enough to create a huge gap between modern society and the traditional knowledge that kept the man alive and well for thousands of years.

Lately, the ancestral wisdom of herbal remedies is coming back gradually, in an informative form in most cases, since the original experience is now forgotten and has to be acquired almost from scratch.

Mint has been reported by Hippocrates, Dioscourides and Plinious [12] as a plant of high pharmaceutical and therapeutic value.

Easier breathing

The expectorant properties of mint, can help with the symptoms of asthma, allergies, colds, bronchitis etc. [13]

Even though, any form of mint remedy could benefit these cases, the inhalation of menthol seems to be the most suitable.

Steam therapy: In a saucepan, boil 2 cups of water. Add a handful of dried mint leaves and flowers. Turn off the fire, lean over the saucepan, cover your head and the saucepan with a thick towel and inhale the steam.

Embrocate with mint oil: In a tablespoon of almond or sesame oil, add 5 drops of peppermint oil. Mix and massage your chest. You can also apply your homemade mint oil.

Nausea

Do you suffer from nausea because of pregnancy, or every time you travel? In any case, peppermint, the magnificent, can save your day. It relaxes the muscles of the digestive system and regulates the function of the stomach.

Dried leaves and flowers of peppermint are the best choice.

Drink a cup of peppermint. If you are pregnant, you better consult your doctor on how many cups and how often you should drink. If you are about to travel, try a cup before you go, and if it is possible have some with you.

Or

Carry a cloth handkerchief scented with mint essential oil.

Ease the pain

Mint can help with many kinds of pain.

Toothache: Chew some mint leaves, or prepare a small portion of mint cataplasm and place it on the aching tooth.

Rheumatisms: Rub mint leaves on joints, or massage with mint oil extract.

A "minty" touch in my kitchen...

In ancient Greece, rubbing the table with mint leaves before eating, was a customary practice.

Mint is widely used, both in pastry and cooking. Specifically, spearmint applies as a flavouring, mostly in meals, and peppermint in desserts and drinks.

Mediterranean cuisine adores and adapts mint in many dishes, as well as in salads, sauces, and oil or vinegar mixtures.

Fresh spearmint leaves are the ultimate ingredient for salads, such as tomato with cucumber, onion, vinegar and olive oil.

Liqueur

I have already mentioned the stimulative effect of the mint aroma, which is caused by the menthol substance. Therefore, mint liqueur is considered an **excellent tonic**, and also, a fine **digestive drink**.

You can definitely find it at the market, however, if you have the time and patience, you can prepare it yourself. The flavour might be less strong, but you'll be absolutely certain that it comes from real and pure mint!

The secret for a successful homemade liqueur is to use a good quality alcohol base.

Ingredients:
1 quart (1lt) of good quality vodka (or Greek Tsipouro)
2 cups of water
1 pound sugar
2 bunches of fresh mint
How to:
Wash the mint and place it on an absorbent towel for a while, to absorb the liquids. Cut all the leaves with your hands and put them in a sterilized jar or bottle; it must have a lid that closes well.

Pour the alcohol in the jar and close the lid. Leave it in a sunny place for 10 days, and remember to shake it slightly once a day.

Then, open the jar, or bottle, add the water and the sugar and close again. Let it under the sun for 30 days this time; **don't forget the daily shaking**.

After one month, strain, once or twice if needed, using a tool cloth. Your homemade mint liqueur is ready. Put it in a stylish glass bottle and serve your friends in any occasion.

Besides the liqueur, you have the option to serve yourself a fine Mojito cocktail!

Put 6-8 fresh peppermint leaves in a tall glass, add 1 tbsp black sugar, 3-4 pieces of lime and crush them with a wooden pestle. Add crushed ice, 1 Oz white rum and fill with soda water. Serve with a straw and fresh peppermint leaves.

Sauce

Making a mint sauce, it's a bit like making... a Mojito cocktail!

Ingredients:
2 handfuls of fresh mint leaves (finely chopped)
1 cup of white wine vinegar (or lemon)
2 tbsp brown sugar
A pinch of salt

How to: Use a pestle to crush the mint leaves and the sugar. Add the vinegar and the salt, and stir until the sugar dissolves completely. Put it in the fridge for a while and serve chilled or warmed, depending on the dish.

Mint sauce is usually combined with meat dishes. However, if you are vegetarian, as me, you can try it with pasta, or replace the vinegar with lemon and combine with mashed potatoes.

Syrup

Would you like a homemade syrup to garnish ice cream, fruit salads, pancakes and tea beverages? The mint syrup is the ideal choice!

Ingredients:
2 handfuls of fresh mint leaves
1 cup of brown sugar
1 cup of water

Use a wooden or ceramic pestle to crush, once again, the mint leaves along with the sugar. In a saucepan, put the water and the mint mixture. Simmer over medium heat, stirring continuously. When the sugar is completely dissolved, and the liquid starts to thicken, remove from fire and let it aside for a while to chill. Then strain and keep it in a sterilized jar in the fridge.

If you want more, double the portions of the ingredients.

Pesto

A nice delicious pesto with a mint flavour, instead of basil!

Ingredients:
1 cup olive oil
2 handfuls of fresh mint leaves
3 garlic cloves
1 tbsp pine seeds
Salt and pepper

How to: Peel and chop the garlic, wash and dry the mint. Put the garlic, the mint leaves and the pine seeds in a bowl, and mash them with a pestle. While you mashing, pour gradually the olive oil and mix well. Season with salt and pepper.

Mix with warm pasta and serve!

Mint, the Miraculous Herb

Mint Varieties

1. Mentha Aquatica
2. **Mentha arvensis syn. Mentha parvifolia:** *It is widespread in the plains and fields.*
3. Mentha asiatica
4. Mentha Australis
5. Mentha Canadensis
6. Mentha cervina
7. Mentha citrate
8. Mentha crispate
9. Mentha cunninghamia
10. Mentha dahurica
11. Mentha diemenica
12. Mentha gattefossei
13. Mentha grandiflora
14. Mentha micrantha
15. Mentha haplocalyx
16. Mentha japonica
17. Mentha kopetdaghensis
18. Mentha laxiflora
19. Mentha longifolia syn. Mentha nigrescens
20. Mentha nemorosa
21. Mentha pubescens
22. **Mentha pulegium:** *Its common name is pennyroyal, vlichoni, fleskouni or vlichouni. It is mainly used for food flavouring and infusions. It is a perennial plant. Its leaves are small and oval and the flowers are pink or purple. The blossoming begins in June and lasts until October.*
23. **Mentha x piperita:** *It has a strong fragrance and a spicy taste. The peppermint is the hybrid of crossing species of Mentha Spicata and Mentha Aquatica. It is a perennial plant and it reaches the height of 80cm. Peppermint leaves are oval - round with a slightly fluffy bottom surface. Its flowers are white or light purple. It is native to humid ground. It blooms from July to September. Better collected when it is in full blooming. From the leaves and the flow-*

ers we get the essential oil which contains menthol and is used in pastry, beverage industry and pharmaceuticals.

24. **Mentha spicata subsp. Spicata or Mentha viridis:** *Spearmint, the Greek "Diosmos" which is widely used for infusions and syrups.*
25. Mentha requienii
26. Mentha x rotundifolia
27. Mentha sachalinensis
28. Mentha satureioides
29. Mentha suaveolens
30. Mentha longifolia var. asiatica / Mentha vagans

*The little x means that this specific variety is a hybrid.

Just a few mint quotes before you go...

"Nothing except the mint can make money without advertising"
Thomas B. Macaulay

"It is the destiny of mint to be crushed"
Waverley Lewis Root

"The mint makes it first, it's up to you to make it last"
Evan Esar

References and Notes

1. Notes on Supplementary Plates CLXXVII-CLXXX.

2. Lamiaceae or Labiatae : Family of flowering plants.

3. Kokytos or Cocytos, the "river of wailing", was one of the five rivers that surrounded Hades.

4. *"Applying a peppermint solution to the skin at the start of a migraine and again 30 minutes later seems to increase the percentage of patients who experience headache resolution."* [U.S. National Library of Medicine]

5. *"In vapor therapy, peppermint oil can help to increase concentration and to stimulate the mind, as well as sorting out coughs, headaches, nausea and also has value as an insect repellant."* [Asian Journal of Pharmaceutical and Clinical Research]

6. *"Peppermint and its EO are believed to be effective in the treatment of nervous disorders and mental fatigue (Tisserand, 1993),suggesting that they may exert some psychoactive actions."* [Asian Journal of Pharmaceutical and Clinical Research]

7. *"Peppermint calms the muscles of the stomach and improves the flow of bile, which the body uses to digest fats. As a result, food passes through the stomach more quickly. However, if your symptoms of indigestion are related to a condition called gastroesophageal reflux disease or GERD, you should not use peppermint"* [Pennstat Hersey Medical Center]

8. *"..Dr Stuart Brierley says while peppermint has been commonly prescribed by naturopaths for many years, there has been no clinical evidence until now to demonstrate why it is so effective in relieving pain. "Our research shows that peppermint acts through a specific anti-pain channel called TRPM8 to reduce pain sensing fibres, particularly those activated by mustard and chilli. This is potentially the first step in determining a new type of mainstream clinical treatment for Irritable Bowel Syndrome (IBS)," he says..."* [Peppermint earns respect in mainstream medicine, The University of Adelaide]

9. *"...110 people with IBS were given either enteric-coated peppermint oil (187 mg) or placebo 3-4 times daily, 15 to 30 minutes before meals, for 4 weeks. 8 The results showed significant improvements in abdominal pain, bloating, stool frequency, and flatulence. In a similar study, people who took peppermint oil capsules for 8 weeks also had less abdominal pain and discomfort compared to the placebo group..."* [NYU Langone Medical Center]

10. Review of Impotence Natural remedies for impotence in medieval Persia, M. Khaleghi Ghadiri and A. Gorji

11. *"one drachma of rock salt - a measure equal to one hundredth of an ounce - two drachmas of mint, one drachma of dried iris flower and 20 grains of pepper, all of them crushed and mixed together."* The recipe, written in Greek, the official language of Egypt for about 1,000 years until the last temples closed in the sixth century AD, was discovered among ancient Egyptian documents such as stone and clay tablets gathered by the Habsburgs, the rulers of the Austro-Hungarian empire. [World's oldest toothpaste formula found on papyrus scroll, GMA News]

12. Hippocrates: ancient Greek physician, philosopher, who is considered the "father of medicine" . Dioscorides: Greek physician, pharmacologist and botanist, who travelled through the Roman Empire, collecting samples of medicinal herbs. Plinius: Roman author, naturalist and natural philosopher.

13. *"According to research published in the July 2010 issue of "Journal of Ethnopharmacology," it was noted that peppermint oil was found to have anti-congestive, antispasmodic (meaning it helps relax the smooth muscles of respiratory tract), and expectorant properties. This study found that 100-300 micrograms of peppermint oil relaxed the trachea in rats."* {Global Healing Center, The Lung Cleansing Benefits of Peppermint, source: Antispasmodic effect of Mentha piperita essential oil on tracheal smooth muscle of rats. J Ethnopharmacol. 2010 Jul 20]

Disclaimer

The above information is a sharing of traditional knowledge and experiences for educational and informational purposes. It does not constitute medical diagnosis or medication recommendation. This book is not intended to substitute professional diagnosis and treatment. Also, is not intended to replace any medication you are already taking or the advice of your doctor.

The author and the publishers disclaim any warranties and are not liable for excessive and careless use, for any incidental or consequential damage connected direct or indirectly with the content of this ebook, or the ignoring of the recommendations of your doctor.

The liability, use, misuse, negligence of any recipe, instruction or ideas given in this book is under the total responsibility of the reader.

Author and publisher disclaim also any warranties for the accuracy of the external links content.

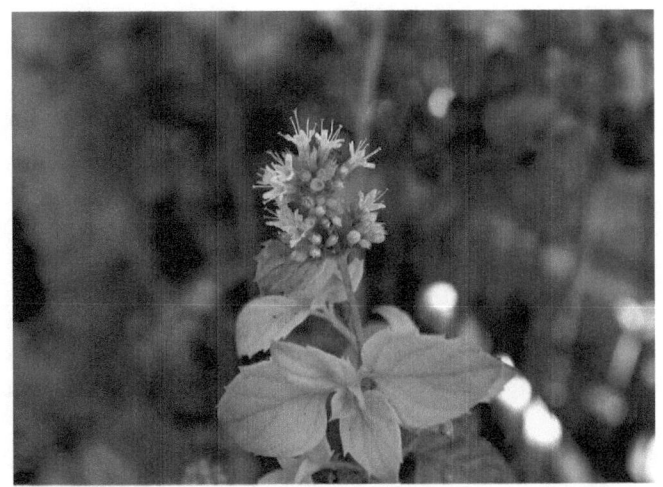

Visit : http://evelinbooks.wordpress.com

for updates, beauty and cooking recipes,
tips and instructions for homemade products,
ideas sharing and lots of colourful images!

Reties

"Reading this very short book is about all you'll need to start grow-
ing mint, if need be, in pots on your window sill.
This is a fabulous little book, telling the history of growing mint.
While it could be expected to find out that the old Romans, Greek and
Medieval monks put mint to good use, I learned new information, for
instance, that the aphrodisiac properties of the plant, have been high-
ly praised since ancient times. In the Arab world, from antiquity until
today, mint and specifically peppermint tea are used to enhance sexu-
al arousal."
[Gisela Hausmann, author and blogger, Review from 1st digital edition]

"This is great I grow different types of mint and this teaches me new
and exciting uses for it a great buy"
[Cindy Jones, Review from 1st digital edition]

Whenever I have had a damp spot that would support mint I have had
a patch. Other than putting in my drink at times I never made full use
of this herb. Even though I live in the desert I will get another patch
going and try these recipes.
[Lindah, Review from 1st digital edition]

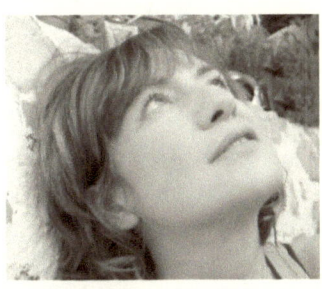

"Hello again!
This my second short guide of one more mi-
raculous herb: The Mint!
People all around the world love this fa-
mous flavour.
I tried to collect the most useful and inter-
esting applications and facts about mint,
and I hope you will find it useful, easy to
read and handy.
Thank you!!"

Mint, the Miraculous Herb